The Mediterranean Diet Cookbook for Beginners

Discover our recipes and improve your life, 50 days of complete and delicious recipes that will help you lose weight and make your life healthier.

Marta Anderson

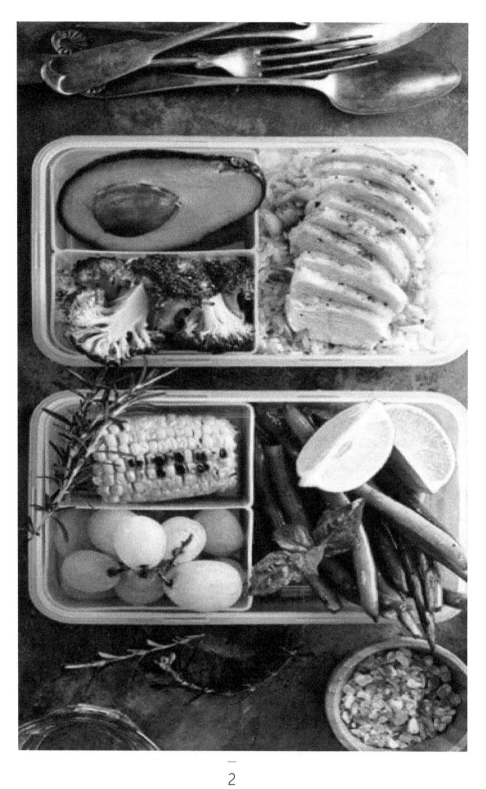

Introduction:

What is Mediterranean Diet?

The Mediterranean Diet is a Diet Inspired by the Eating Habits of Spain, Italy, and Greece in the 1960s. In this Book you will Find Everything You Need to Cook Healthy and Delicious Recipes. All the Ingredients will be Easy to Find and You will be Followed Step By Step for the Realization of the Recipes

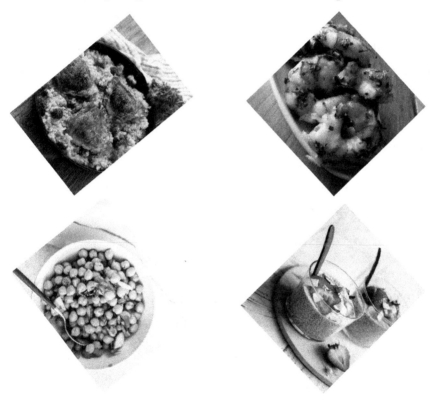

Table of Contents

Snacks

Spinach Artichoke-stuffed Chicken Breasts

Preparation Time: 15 Minutes

Cooking Time: 15 Minutes

Servings: 6

Ingredients:

- ¼ cup Greek yogurt

- ¼ cup spinach, thawed & drained

- ½ cup artichoke hearts, thinly sliced

- ½ cup mozzarella cheese, shredded

- 1 ½ lb. chicken breasts

- 2 tablespoons. olive oil

- 4 ozs. cream cheese

- Sea salt & pepper, to taste

Directions:

1. Pound the chicken breasts to a thickness of about one inch. Using a sharp knife, slice a "pocket" into the side of each. This is where you will put the filling.

2. Sprinkle the breasts with salt and pepper and set aside.

3. In a medium bowl, combine cream cheese, yogurt, mozzarella, spinach, artichoke, salt, and pepper and mix thoroughly. A hand mixer may be the easiest way to combine all the ingredients thoroughly.

4. Spoon the mixture into the pockets of each breast and set aside while you heat a large skillet over medium heat and warm the oil in it. If you have an extra filling you can't fit into the breasts, set it aside until just before your chicken is done cooking.

5. Cook each breast for about eight minutes per side, then pull off the heat when it reaches an internal temperature of about 165° Fahrenheit.

6. Just before you pull the chicken out of the pan, heat the remaining filling to warm it through and to rid it of any cross-contamination from the chicken. Once hot, top the chicken breasts with it.

7. Serve!

Nutrition:

- Calories: 238

- Fat: 22 g

- Carbs: 5 g

- Protein: 17 g

- Fiber: 4 g

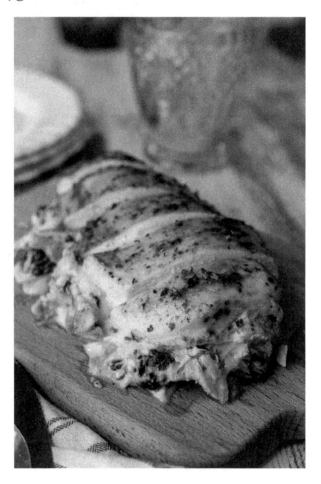

Chicken Parmesan

Preparation Time: 20 Minutes

Cooking Time: 15 Minutes

Servings: 4

Ingredients:

- ¼ cup of avocado oil

- ¼ cup of almond flour

- ¼ cup parmesan cheese, grated

- ¾ cup of marinara sauce, sugar-free

- ¾ cup mozzarella cheese, shredded

- 2 eggs, beaten

- 2 teaspoons. Italian seasoning

- 3 oz. pork rinds, pulverized

- 4 lbs. chicken breasts, boneless & skinless

- Sea salt & pepper, to taste

Directions:

1. Preheat the oven to 450° Fahrenheit and grease a baking dish.

2. Place the beaten egg into one shallow dish. Place the almond flour in another. In a third dish, combine the pork rinds, parmesan, and Italian seasoning and mix well.

3. Pat the chicken breasts dry and pound them down to about ½" thick.

4. Dredge the chicken in the almond flour, then coat in egg, then coat in crumb.

5. Heat a large sauté pan over medium-high heat and warm oil until shimmering.

6. Once the oil is hot, lay the breasts into the pan and do not move them until they've had a chance to cook. Cook for about two minutes, then flip as gently as possible (a fish spatula is perfect) then cook for two more. Remove the pan from the heat.

7. Place the breasts in the greased baking dish and top with marinara sauce and mozzarella cheese.

8. Bake for about 10 minutes.

9. Serve!

Nutrition:

- Calories: 621

- Fat: 24 g

- Carbs: 6 g

- Protein: 14 g

- Fiber: 6 g

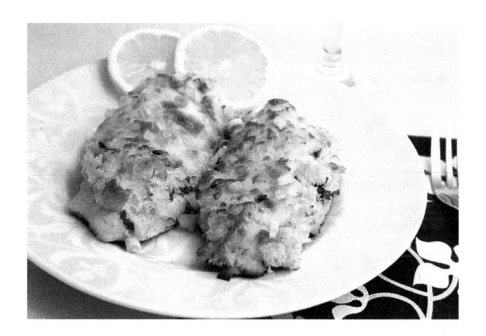

Sheet Pan Jalapeño Burgers

Preparation Time: 10 Minutes

Cooking Time: 20 Minutes

Servings: 4

Ingredients:

Burgers:

- 24 ozs. ground beef

- Sea salt & pepper, to taste

- ½ teaspoon. garlic powder

- 6 slices bacon, halved

- 1 med. onion, sliced into ¼ rounds

- 2 jalapeños, seeded & sliced

- 4 slices pepper jack cheese

- ¼ cup of mayonnaise

- 1 tablespoon. chili sauce

- ½ teaspoon. Worcestershire sauce

- 8 lbs. leaves of Boston or butter lettuce

- 8 dill pickle chips

Directions:

1. Preheat the oven to 425° Fahrenheit and line a baking sheet with non-stick foil.

2. Mix the salt, pepper, and garlic into the ground beef and form 4 patties out of it.

3. Line the burgers, bacon slices, jalapeño slices, and onion rounds onto the baking sheet and bake for about 18 minutes.

4. Top each patty with a piece of cheese and set the oven to boil.

5. Broil for 2 minutes, then remove the pan from the oven.

6. Serve one patty with 3 pieces of bacon, jalapeño slices, onion rounds, and desired amount of sauce with 2 pickle chips and 2 parts of lettuce.

7. Enjoy!

Nutrition:

- Calories: 608

- Fat: 29 g

- Carbs: 5 g

- Protein: 16 g

- Fiber: 4 g

Grilled Herb Garlic Chicken

Preparation Time: 5 Minutes

Cooking Time: 10 Minutes

Servings: 2

Ingredients:

- 1 ¼ lb. chicken breasts, boneless & skinless - 1 tablespoon. garlic & herb seasoning mix

- 2 teaspoons. extra virgin olive oil - Sea salt & pepper, to taste

Directions:

1. Heat a grill pan or your grill.

2. Coat the chicken breasts in a little bit of olive oil and then sprinkle the seasoning mixture onto them, rubbing it in.

3. Cook the chicken for about eight minutes per side and make sure the chicken has reached an internal temperature of 165°.

4. Serve hot with your favorite sides!

Nutrition:

- Calories: 187

- Fat: 24 g

- Carbs: 5 g

- Protein: 12 g

- Fiber: 4 g

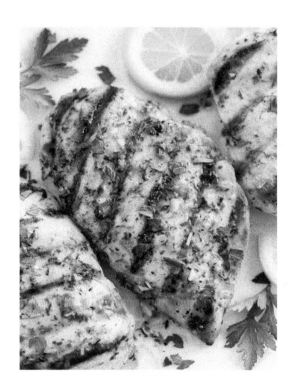

Blackened Salmon with Avocado Salsa

Preparation Time: 30 Minutes

Cooking Time: 21 Minutes

Servings: 6

Ingredients:

- 1 tablespoon. extra virgin olive oil

- 4 filets of salmon (about 6 ozs. each)

- 4 teaspoons. Cajun seasoning

- 2 med. avocados, diced

- 1 cup cucumber, diced

- ¼ cup red onion, diced

- 1 tablespoon. parsley, chopped

- 1 tablespoon. lime juice

- Sea salt & pepper, to taste

Directions:

1. Heat a skillet over medium-high heat and warm the oil in it.

2. Rub the Cajun seasoning into the fillets, then lay them into the bottom of the skillet once it's hot enough.

3. Cook until a dark crust forms, then flip and repeat.

4. In a medium mixing bowl, combine all the ingredients for the salsa and set aside.

5. Plate the fillets and top with ¼ of the salsa yielded.

6. Enjoy!

Nutrition:

- Calories: 445

- Fat: 31 g

- Carbs: 6 g

- Protein: 10 g

- Fiber: 5 g

Lean and Green

Pesto Zucchini Noodles

Preparation Time: 15 minutes

Cooking Time: minutes 15 minutes

Servings: 4

Ingredients:

- 4 zucchini, spiralized
- 1 tbsp avocado oil
- 2 garlic cloves, chopped
- 2/3 cup olive oil
- 1/3 cup parmesan cheese, grated
- 2 cups fresh basil
- 1/3 cup almonds
- 1/8 tsp black pepper
- ¾ tsp sea salt

Directions:

1. Add zucchini noodles into a colander and sprinkle with ¼ teaspoon of salt. Cover and let sit for 30 minutes. Drain zucchini noodles well and pat dry.

2. Preheat the oven to 400 F.

3. Place almonds on a parchment-lined baking sheet and bake for 6-8 minutes.

4. Transfer toasted almonds into the food processor and process until coarse.

5. Add olive oil, cheese, basil, garlic, pepper, and remaining salt in a food processor with almonds and process until pesto texture.

6. Heat avocado oil in a large pan over medium-high heat.

7. Add zucchini noodles and cook for 4-5 minutes.

8. Pour pesto over zucchini noodles, mix well and cook for 1 minute.

9. Serve immediately with baked salmon.

Nutrition:

Calories: 525

Fat 44 g

Carbs 3 g

Sugar 8 g

Protein 16 g

Cholesterol 30 mg

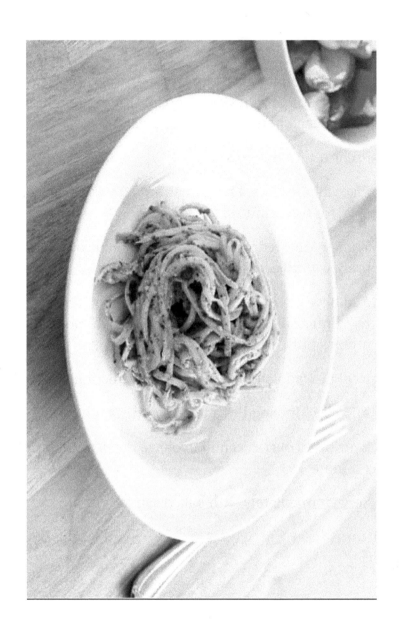

Baked Cod & Vegetables

Preparation Time: 15 minutes

Cooking Time: 15 minutes

Servings: 4

Ingredients:

- 1 lb cod fillets

- 8 oz asparagus, chopped

- 3 cups broccoli, chopped

- ¼ cup parsley, minced

- ½ tsp lemon pepper seasoning

- ½ tsp paprika

- ¼ cup olive oil

- ¼ cup lemon juice

- 1 tsp salt

Directions:

1. Preheat oven to 400 F. Line a baking sheet with parchment paper and set aside.

2. In a small bowl, combine the lemon juice, paprika, olive oil, pepper spices, and salt.

3. Place the fish fillets in the center of the greaseproof paper. Arrange the broccoli and asparagus around the fish fillets.

4. Pour lemon juice mixture over the fish fillets and top with parsley.

5. Bake in preheated oven for 13-15 minutes.

6. Serve and enjoy.

Nutrition:

Calories: 240

Fat: 11 g

Carbs: 6 g

Sugar: 6 g

Protein: 27 g

Cholesterol: 56 mg

Parmesan Zucchini

Preparation Time: 15 minutes

Cooking Time: 15 minutes

Servings: 4

Ingredients:

- 4 zucchini, quartered lengthwise
- 2 tbsp fresh parsley, chopped
- 2 tbsp olive oil
- ¼ tsp garlic powder
- ½ tsp dried basil
- ½ tsp dried oregano
- ½ tsp dried thyme
- ½ cup parmesan cheese, grated
- Pepper
- Salt

Directions:

1. Preheat the oven to 350 F. Line baking sheet with parchment paper and set aside.

2. In a small bowl, mix together parmesan cheese, garlic powder, basil, oregano, thyme, pepper, and salt.

3. Arrange zucchini onto the prepared baking sheet and drizzle with oil and sprinkle with parmesan cheese mixture.

4. Bake in preheated oven for 15 minutes then broil for 2 minutes or until lightly golden brown.

5. Garnish with parsley and serve immediately.

Nutrition:

Calories: 244

Fat: 14 g

Carbs: 7 g

Sugar: 5 g

Protein: 15 g

Cholesterol: 30 mg

Chicken Zucchini Noodles

Preparation Time: 20 minutes

Cooking Time: 5 minutes

Servings: 2

Ingredients:

- 1 large zucchini, spiralized
- 1 chicken breast, skinless & boneless
- ½ tbsp jalapeno, minced
- 2 garlic cloves, minced
- ½ tsp ginger, minced
- ½ tbsp fish sauce
- 2 tbsp coconut cream
- ½ tbsp honey
- ½ lime juice
- 1 tbsp peanut butter
- 1 carrot, chopped
- 2 tbsp cashews, chopped
- ¼ cup fresh cilantro, chopped
- 1 tbsp olive oil
- Pepper

- Salt

Directions:

1. Heat olive oil in a pan over medium-high heat.

2. Season chicken breast with pepper and salt. Once the oil is hot then add chicken breast into the pan and cook for 3-4 minutes per side or until cooked.

3. Remove chicken breast from pan. Shred chicken breast with a fork and set aside.

4. In a small bowl, mix together peanut butter, jalapeno, garlic, ginger, fish sauce, coconut cream, honey, and lime juice. Set aside.

5. In a large mixing bowl, combine together spiralized zucchini, carrots, cashews, cilantro, and shredded chicken.

6. Pour peanut butter mixture over zucchini noodles and toss to combine.

7. Serve immediately and enjoy.

Nutrition:

Calories 353

Fat 21 g

Carbs 20.5 g

Sugar 8 g

Protein 25 g

Cholesterol 54 mg

Tomato Cucumber Avocado Salad

Preparation Time: 15 minutes

Cooking Time: 0 minutes

Servings: 4

Ingredients:

- 12 oz cherry tomatoes, cut in half

- 5 small cucumbers, chopped

- 3 small avocados, chopped

- ½ tsp ground black pepper

- 2 tbsp olive oil

- 2 tbsp fresh lemon juice

- ¼ cup fresh cilantro, chopped

- 1 tsp sea salt

Directions:

1. Add cherry tomatoes, cucumbers, avocados, and cilantro into the large mixing bowl and mix well.

2. Mix together olive oil, lemon juice, black pepper, and salt and pour over salad.

3. Toss well and serve immediately.

Nutrition:

Calories: 442

Fat: 31 g

Carbs: 30.3 g

Sugar: 4 g

Protein: 2 g

Cholesterol: 0 mg

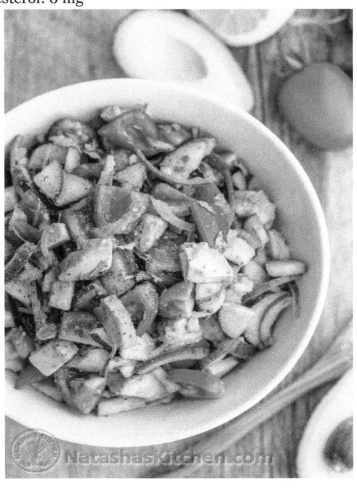

Salad

Barb's Asian Slaw

Preparation Time: 5 minutes

Cooking Time: 5 minutes

Servings: 2

Ingredients:

- 1 cabbage head, shredded

- 4 chopped green onions

- ½ cup slivered or sliced almonds

Dressing:

- ½ cup olive oil

- ¼ cup tamari or soy sauce

- 1 tablespoon honey or maple syrup

- 1 tablespoon baking stevia

Directions:

1. Heat up dressing ingredients in a saucepan on the stove until thoroughly mixed.

2. Mix all ingredients when you are ready to serve.

Nutrition:

Calories: 205

Protein: 27g

Carbohydrate: 12g

Fat: 10 g

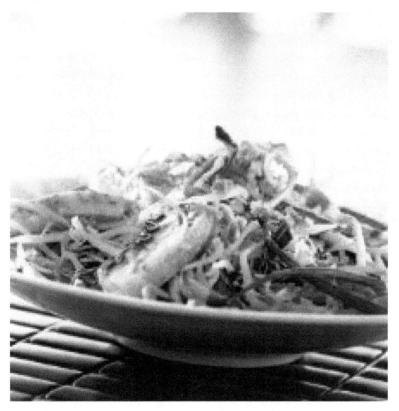

Blueberry Cantaloupe Avocado Salad

Preparation Time: 5 minutes

Cooking Time: 0 minutes

Servings: 2

Ingredients:

- 1 diced cantaloupe

- 2–3 chopped avocados

- 1 package of blueberries

- ¼ cup olive oil

- 1/8 cup balsamic vinegar

Directions:

1. Mix all ingredients.

Nutrition:

Calories: 406

Protein: 9g

Carbohydrate: 32g

Fat: 5g

Beet Salad (from Israel)

Preparation Time: 5 minutes

Cooking Time: 0 minutes

Servings: 2

Ingredients:

- 2–3 fresh, raw beets grated or shredded in food processor
- 3 tablespoons olive oil
- 2 tablespoons balsamic vinegar
- ¼ teaspoon salt
- 1/3 teaspoon cumin
- Dash stevia powder or liquid
- Dash pepper

Directions:

1. Mix all ingredients together for the best raw beet salad.

Nutrition:

Calories: 156

Protein: 8g

Carbohydrate: 40g

Fat: 5 g

Broccoli Salad

Preparation Time: 5 minutes

Cooking Time: 0 minutes

Servings: 2

Ingredients:

- 1 head broccoli, chopped
- 2–3 slices of fried bacon, crumbled
- 1 diced green onion
- ½ cup raisins or craisins
- ½–1 cup of chopped pecans
- ¾ cup sunflower seeds
- ½ cup of pomegranate

Dressing:

- 1 cup organic mayonnaise
- ¼ cup baking stevia
- 2 teaspoons white vinegar

Directions:

1. Mix all ingredients together. Mix dressing and fold into salad.

Nutrition:

Calories: 239

Protein: 10g

Carbohydrate: 33g

Fat: 2g

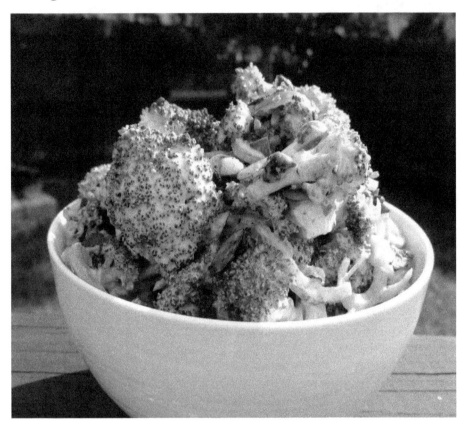

Roasted Garlic Potatoes

Preparation Time: 5 minutes

Cooking Time: 30 minutes

Servings: 2

Ingredients:

- 5 red new potatoes, chopped

- ¼ cup olive oil

- 2–3 cloves of minced garlic

- 1 tablespoon rosemary

Directions:

1. Preheat oven to 425 degrees.

2. Stir all ingredients together in a bowl. Pour onto a baking sheet and bake for 30 minutes.

Nutrition:

Calories: 176

Protein: 5g

Carbohydrate: 30g

Fat: 2g

Poultry

Country-Style Chicken Stew

Preparation Time: 20 minutes

Cooking Time: 1 hour

Servings: 6

Ingredients:

- 1 pound chicken thighs
- 2 tablespoons butter, room temperature
- 1/2 pound carrots, chopped
- 1 bell pepper, chopped
- 1 chile pepper, deveined and minced
- 1 cup tomato puree
- Kosher salt and ground black pepper, to taste
- 1/2 teaspoon smoked paprika
- 1 onion, finely chopped
- 1 teaspoon garlic, sliced
- 4 cups vegetable broth
- 1 teaspoon dried basil

- 1 celery, chopped

Directions:

1. Melt the butter in a stockpot over medium-high flame. Sweat the onion and garlic until just tender and fragrant.

2. Reduce the heat to medium-low. Stir in the broth, chicken thighs, and basil; bring to a rolling boil.

3. Add in the remaining Ingredients. Partially cover and let it simmer for 45 to 50 minutes. Shred the meat, discarding the bones; add the chicken back to the pot.

Nutrition:

Calories: 280

Fat: 14.7g

Carbs: 2.5g

Protein: 25.6g

Fiber: 2.5g

Autumn Chicken Soup with Root Vegetables

Preparation Time: 10 minutes

Cooking Time: 25 minutes

Servings: 4

Ingredients:

- 4 cups chicken broth
- 1 cup full-fat milk
- 1 cup double cream
- 1/2 cup turnip, chopped
- 2 chicken drumsticks, boneless and cut into small pieces
- Salt and pepper, to taste
- 1 tablespoon butter
- 1 teaspoon garlic, finely minced
- 1 carrot, chopped
- 1/2 parsnip, chopped
- 1/2 celery
- 1 whole egg

Directions:

1. Melt the butter in a heavy-bottomed pot over medium-high heat; sauté the garlic until aromatic or about 1 minute. Add in the vegetables and continue to cook until they've softened.

2. Add in the chicken and cook until it is no longer pink for about 4 minutes. Season with salt and pepper.

3. Pour in the chicken broth, milk, and heavy cream and bring it to a boil.

4. Reduce the heat to. Partially cover and continue to simmer for 20 to 25 minutes longer. Afterwards, fold the beaten egg and stir until it is well incorporated.

Nutrition:

Calories: 342

Fat: 22.4g

Carbs: 6.3g

Protein: 25.2g

Fiber: 1.3g

Panna Cotta with Chicken and Bleu d' Auvergne

Preparation Time: 10 minutes

Cooking Time: 20 minutes

Servings:

Ingredients:

- 2 chicken legs, boneless and skinless

- 1 tablespoon avocado oil

- 2 teaspoons granular erythritol

- 3 tablespoons water

- 1 cup Bleu d' Auvergne, crumbled

- 2 gelatin sheets

- 3/4 cup double cream

- Salt and cayenne pepper, to your liking

Directions:

1. Heat the oil in a frying pan over medium-high heat; fry the chicken for about 10 minutes.

2. Soak the gelatin sheets in cold water. Cook with the cream, erythritol, water, and Bleu d' Auvergne.

3. Season with salt and pepper and let it simmer over the low heat, stirring for about 3 minutes. Spoon the mixture into four ramekins.

Nutrition:

Calories: 306

Fat: 18.3g

Carbs. 4.7g

Protein: 29.5g

Fiber: 0g

Breaded Chicken Fillets

Preparation Time: 15 minutes

Cooking Time: 30 minutes

Servings: 4

Ingredients:

- 1 pound chicken fillets
- 3 bell peppers, quartered lengthwise
- 1/3 cup Romano cheese
- 2 teaspoons olive oil
- 1 garlic clove, minced
- Kosher salt and ground black pepper, to taste
- 1/3 cup crushed pork rinds

Directions:

1. Start by preheating your oven to 410 degrees F.

2. Mix the crushed pork rinds, Romano cheese, olive oil and minced garlic. Dredge the chicken into this mixture.

3. Place the chicken in a lightly greased baking dish. Season with salt and black pepper to taste.

4. Scatter the peppers around the chicken and bake in the preheated oven for 20 to 25 minutes or until thoroughly cooked.

Nutrition:

Calories: 367

Fat: 16.9g

Carbs: 6g

Protein: 43g

Fiber: 0.7g

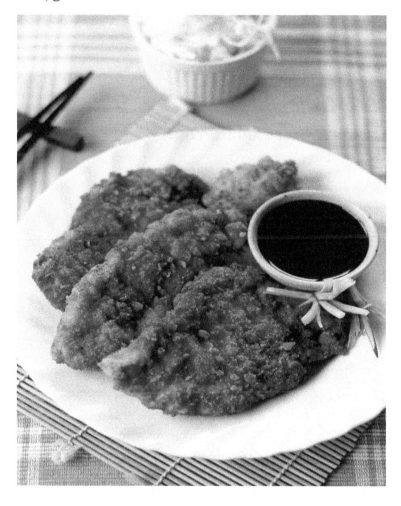

Chicken Drumsticks with Broccoli and Cheese

Preparation Time: 40 minutes

Cooking Time: 1 hour 15 minutes

Servings: 4

Ingredients:

- 1 pound chicken drumsticks

- 1 pound broccoli, broken into florets

- 2 cups cheddar cheese, shredded

- 1/2 teaspoon dried oregano

- 1/2 teaspoon dried basil

- 3 tablespoons olive oil

- 1 celery, sliced

- 1 cup green onions, chopped

- 1 teaspoon minced green garlic

Directions:

1. Roast the chicken drumsticks in the preheated oven at 380 degrees F for 30 to 35 minutes. Add in the broccoli, celery, green onions, and green garlic.

2. Add in the oregano, basil and olive oil; roast an additional 15 minutes.

Nutrition:

Calories: 533

Fat: 40.2g

Carbs: 5.4g

Protein: 35.1g

Fiber: 3.5g

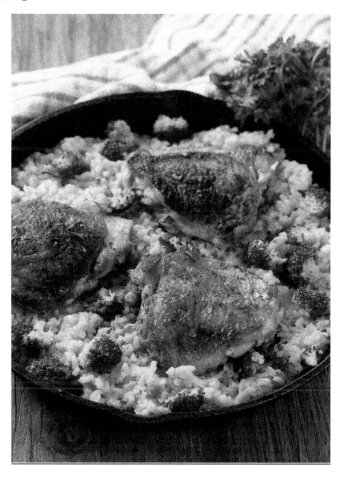

Meat

Beef & Cheddar Stuffed Eggplants

Preparation Time: 15 minutes

Cooking Time: 30 minutes

Servings: 4

Ingredients:

- 2 eggplants
- 2 tbsp olive oil
- 1 ½ lb ground beef
- 1 medium red onion, chopped
- 1 roasted red pepper, chopped
- Pink salt and black pepper to taste
- 1 cup yellow cheddar cheese, grated
- 2 tbsp dill, chopped

Directions:

1. Preheat oven to 350°F. Lay the eggplants on a flat surface, trim off the ends, and cut in half lengthwise. Scoop out the pulp from each half to make shells. Chop the pulp. Heat oil in a skillet over medium heat. Add the ground beef, red onion, pimiento, and eggplant pulp and season with salt and pepper.

2. Cook for 6 minutes while stirring to break up lumps until beef is no longer pink. Spoon the beef into the eggplant shells and sprinkle with cheddar cheese. Place on a greased baking sheet and cook to melt the cheese for 15 minutes until eggplant is tender. Serve warm topped with dill.

Nutrition:

Calories: 574

Fat: 27.5g

Carbs: 9.8g

Protein: 61,8g

Sweet Chipotle Grilled Beef Ribs

Preparation Time: 10 minutes

Cooking Time: 35 minutes

Servings: 4

Ingredients:

- 4 tbsp sugar-free BBQ sauce + extra for serving
- 2 tbsp erythritol
- Pink salt and black pepper to taste
- 2 tbsp olive oil
- 2 tsp chipotle powder
- 1 tsp garlic powder
- 1 lb beef spare ribs

Directions:

1. Mix the erythritol, salt, pepper, oil, chipotle, and garlic powder. Brush on the meaty sides of the ribs and wrap in foil. Sit for 30 minutes to marinate.

2. Preheat oven to 400°F. Place wrapped ribs on a baking sheet and cook for 40 minutes until cooked through.

3. Remove ribs and aluminium foil, brush with BBQ sauce, and brown under the broiler for 10 minutes on both sides. Slice and serve with extra BBQ sauce and lettuce tomato salad.

Nutrition:

Calories: 395

Fat: 33g

Carbs: 3g

Protein: 21g

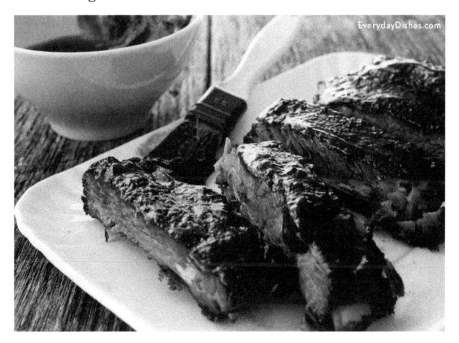

Grilled Sirloin Steak with Sauce Diane

Preparation Time: 10 minutes

Cooking Time: 25 minutes

Servings: 6

Ingredients:

- Sirloin steak

- 1 ½ lb sirloin steak

- Salt and black pepper to taste

- 1 tsp olive oil

- Sauce Diane

- 1 tbsp olive oil

- 1 clove garlic, minced

- 1 cup sliced porcini mushrooms

- 1 small onion, finely diced

- 2 tbsp butter

- 1 tbsp Dijon mustard

- 2 tbsp Worcestershire sauce

- ¼ cup whiskey

- 2 cups heavy cream

Directions:

1. Put a grill pan over high heat and as it heats, brush the steak with oil, sprinkle with salt and pepper, and rub the seasoning into the meat with your hands. Cook the steak in the pan for 4 minutes on each side for medium-rare and transfer to a chopping board to rest for 4 minutes before slicing. Reserve the juice.

2. Heat the oil in a frying pan over medium heat and sauté the onion for 3 minutes. Add the butter, garlic, and mushrooms, and cook for 2 minutes. Add the Worcestershire sauce, the reserved juice, and mustard.

3. Stir and cook for 1 minute. Pour in the whiskey and cook further 1 minute until the sauce reduces by half. Swirl the pan and add the cream. Let it simmer to thicken for about 3 minutes. Adjust the taste with salt and pepper. Spoon the sauce over the steaks slices and serve with celeriac mash.

Nutrition:

Calories: 434

Fat: 17g

Carbs: 2.9g

Protein: 36g

Easy Zucchini Beef Lasagna

Preparation Time: 25 minutes

Cooking Time: 1 hour

Servings: 4

Ingredients:

- 1 lb ground beef
- 2 large zucchinis, sliced lengthwise
- 3 cloves garlic
- 1 medium white onion, chopped
- 3 tomatoes, chopped
- Salt and black pepper to taste
- 2 tsp sweet paprika
- 1 tsp dried thyme
- 1 tsp dried basil
- 1 cup mozzarella cheese, shredded
- 1 tbsp olive oil

Directions:

1. Preheat the oven to 370°F. Heat the olive oil in a skillet over medium heat. Cook the beef for 4 minutes while breaking any lumps as you stir.

2. Top with onion, garlic, tomatoes, salt, paprika, and pepper. Stir and continue cooking for 5 minutes.

3. Lay 1/3 of the zucchini slices in the baking dish.

4. Top with 1/3 of the beef mixture and repeat the layering process two more times with the same quantities. Season with basil and thyme. Sprinkle the mozzarella cheese on top and tuck the baking dish in the oven. Bake for 35 minutes.

5. Remove the lasagna and let it rest for 10 minutes before serving.

Nutrition:

Calories: 344

Fat: 17.8g

Carbs: 2.9g

Protein: 40.4g

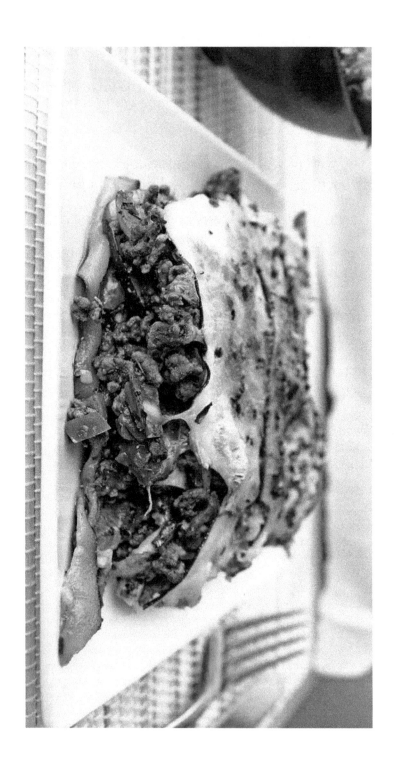

Rib Roast with Roasted Shallots & Garlic

Preparation Time: 15 minutes

Cooking Time: 40 minutes

Servings: 6

Ingredients:

- 5 lb beef rib roast, on the bone

- 3 heads garlic, cut in half

- 3 tbsp olive oil

- 6 shallots, peeled and halved

- 2 lemons, zested and juiced

- 3 tbsp mustard seeds

- 3 tbsp swerve

- Salt and black pepper to taste

- 3 tbsp thyme leaves

Directions:

1. Preheat oven to 400°F. Place garlic heads and shallots in a roasting dish, toss with olive oil, and bake for 15 minutes. Pour lemon juice on them. Score shallow crisscrosses patterns on the meat and set aside.

2. Mix swerve, mustard seeds, thyme, salt, pepper, and lemon zest to make a rub and apply it all over the beef. Place the beef on the shallots and garlic and cook in the oven for 20 minutes. Once ready, remove the dish, and let sit covered for 15 minutes before slicing. Serve.

Nutrition:

Calories: 222

Fat: 29.7g

Carb: 3g,

Protein: 5g

Seafood

Shrimp with Garlic

Preparation Time: 10 minutes

Cooking Time: 25 minutes

Servings: 2

Ingredients:

- 1 lb. shrimp
- ¼ teaspoon baking soda
- 2 tablespoons oil
- 2 teaspoon minced garlic
- ¼ cup vermouth
- 2 tablespoons unsalted butter
- 1 teaspoon parsley

Directions:

1. In a bowl toss shrimp with baking soda and salt, let it stand for a couple of minutes
2. In a skillet heat olive oil and add shrimp
3. Add garlic, red pepper flakes and cook for 1-2 minutes
4. Add vermouth and cook for another 4-5 minutes
5. When ready remove from heat and serve

Nutrition:

Calories: 289

Total Carbohydrate: 2 g

Cholesterol: 3 mg

Total Fat: 17 g

Fiber: 2 g

Protein: 7 g

Sodium: 163 mg

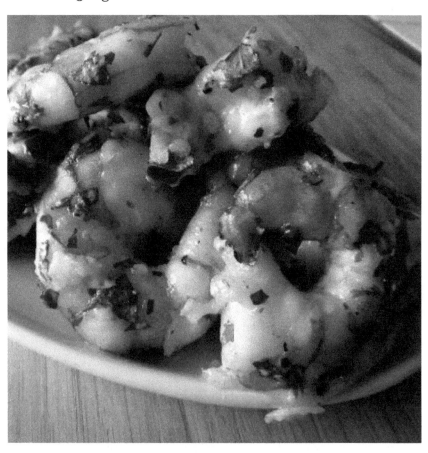

Sabich Sandwich

Preparation Time: 5 minutes

Cooking Time: 15 minutes

Servings: 2

Ingredients:

- 2 tomatoes
- Olive oil
- ½ lb. eggplant
- ¼ cucumber
- 1 tablespoon lemon
- 1 tablespoon parsley
- ¼ head cabbage
- 2 tablespoons wine vinegar
- 2 pita bread
- ½ cup hummus
- ¼ tahini sauce
- 2 hard-boiled eggs

Directions:

1. In a skillet fry eggplant slices until tender

2. In a bowl add tomatoes, cucumber, parsley, lemon juice and season salad

3. In another bowl toss cabbage with vinegar

4. In each pita pocket add hummus, eggplant and drizzle tahini sauce

5. Top with eggs, tahini sauce

Nutrition:

Calories: 269

Total Carbohydrate: 2 g

Cholesterol: 3 mg

Total Fat: 14 g

Fiber: 2 g

Protein: 7 g

Sodium: 183 mg

Salmon with Vegetables

Preparation Time: 10 minutes

Cooking Time: 15 minutes

Servings: 4

Ingredients:

- 2 tablespoons olive oil
- 2 carrots
- 1 head fennel
- 2 squash
- ¼ onion
- 1-inch ginger
- 1 cup white wine
- 2 cups water
- 2 parsley sprigs
- 2 tarragon sprigs
- 6 oz. salmon fillets
- 1 cup cherry tomatoes
- 1 scallion

Directions:

1. In a skillet heat olive oil, add fennel, squash, onion, ginger, carrot and cook until vegetables are soft

2. Add wine, water, parsley and cook for another 4-5 minutes

3. Season salmon fillets and place in the pan

4. Cook for 5 minutes per side or until is ready

5. Transfer salmon to a bowl, spoon tomatoes and scallion around salmon and serve

Nutrition:

Calories: 301

Total Carbohydrate: 2 g

Cholesterol: 13 mg

Total Fat: 17 g

Fiber: 4 g

Protein: 8 g

Sodium: 201 mg

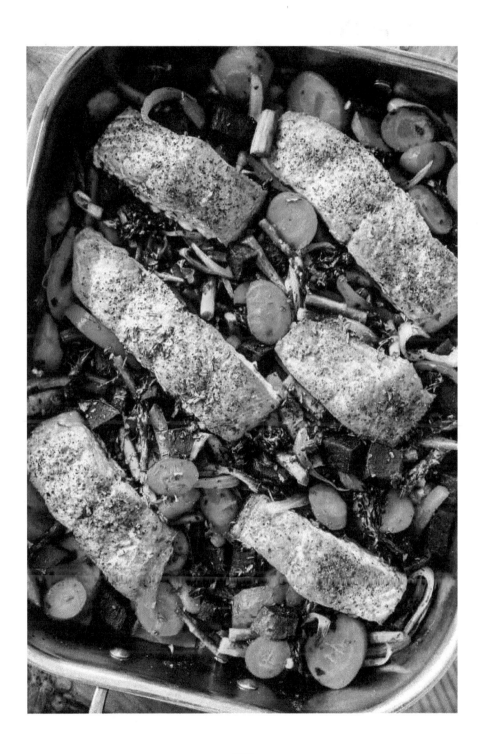

Crispy Fish

Preparation Time: 5 minutes

Cooking Time: 15 minutes

Servings: 4

Ingredients:

- Thick fish fillets
- ¼ cup all-purpose flour
- 1 egg
- 1 cup bread crumbs
- 2 tablespoons vegetables
- Lemon wedge

Directions:

1. In a dish add flour, egg, breadcrumbs in different dishes and set aside

2. Dip each fish fillet into the flour, egg and then bread crumbs bowl

3. Place each fish fillet in a heated skillet and cook for 4-5 minutes per side

4. When ready remove from pan and serve with lemon wedges

Nutrition:

Calories: 189

Total Carbohydrate: 2 g

Cholesterol: 73 mg

Total Fat: 17 g

Fiber: 0 g

Protein: 7 g

Sodium: 163 mg

Moules Marinieres

Preparation Time: 10 minutes

Cooking Time: 30 minutes

Servings: 4

Ingredients:

- 2 tablespoons unsalted butter

- 1 leek

- 1 shallot

- 2 cloves garlic

- 2 bay leaves

- 1 cup white win

- 2 lb. mussels

- 2 tablespoons mayonnaise

- 1 tablespoon lemon zest

- 2 tablespoons parsley

- 1 sourdough bread

Directions:

1. In a saucepan melt butter, add leeks, garlic, bay leaves, shallot and cook until vegetables are soft

2. Bring to a boil, add mussels, and cook for 1-2 minutes

3. Transfer mussels to a bowl and cover

4. Whisk in remaining butter with mayonnaise and return mussels to pot

5. Add lemon juice, parsley lemon zest and stir to combine

Nutrition:

Calories: 321

Total Carbohydrate: 2 g

Cholesterol: 13 mg

Total Fat: 17 g

Fiber: 2 g

Protein: 9 g

Sodium: 312 mg

Sides

Parsley Zucchini and Radishes

> **Preparation time**: 5 minutes
>
> **Cooking time**: 15 minutes
>
> **Servings**: 4

Ingredients:

- 1 pound zucchinis, cubed

- 1 cup radishes, halved

- 1 tablespoon olive oil

- 1 tablespoon balsamic vinegar

- 2 tomatoes, cubed

- 3 tablespoons parsley, chopped

- Salt and black pepper to the taste

Directions:

1. In a pan that fits your air fryer, mix the zucchinis with the radishes, oil and the other ingredients, toss, introduce in the fryer and cook at 350 degrees F for 15 minutes.

2. Divide between plates and serve as a side dish.

Nutrition:

Calories: 170

Fat: 6

Fiber: 2

Carbs: 5

Protein: 6

Cherry Tomatoes Sauté

Preparation time: 5 minutes

Cooking time: 15 minutes

Servings: 4

Ingredients:

- 1 tablespoon olive oil

- 1 pound cherry tomatoes, halved

- Juice of 1 lime

- 2 tablespoons parsley, chopped

- A pinch of salt and black pepper

Directions:

1. In a pan that fits the air fryer, mix the tomatoes with the oil and the other ingredients, toss, introduce the pan in the machine and cook at 360 degrees F for 15 minutes.

2. Divide between plates and serve.

Nutrition:

Calories: 141

Fat: 6

Fiber: 2

Carbs: 4

Protein: 7

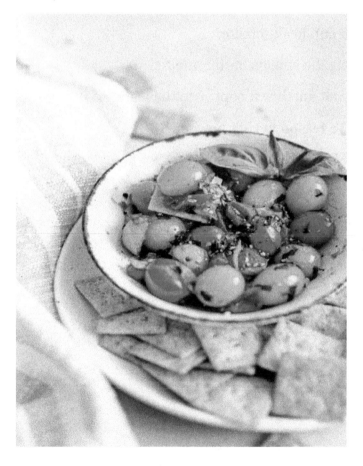

Creamy Eggplant

Preparation time: 5 minutes

Cooking time: 20 minutes

Servings: 4

Ingredients:

 2 pounds eggplants, roughly cubed

 1 cup heavy cream

 2 tablespoons butter, melted

 Salt and black pepper to the taste

 ½ teaspoon chili powder

 ½ teaspoon turmeric powder

Directions:

1. In a pan that fits the air fryer, mix the eggplants with the cream, butter and the other ingredients, toss, introduce in the machine and cook at 370 degrees F for 20 minutes.

2. Divide between plates and serve as a side dish.

Nutrition:

Calories: 151

Fat: 3g

Fiber: 2g

Carbs: 4g

Protein: 6g

Eggplant and Carrots Mix

Preparation time: 5 minutes

Cooking time: 25 minutes

Servings: 4

Ingredients:

- 1 pound eggplants, roughly cubed

- 1 pound baby carrots

- 1 cup heavy cream

- ½ teaspoon chili powder

- 1 teaspoon garlic powder

- 1 tablespoon chives, chopped

- A pinch of salt and black pepper

Directions:

1. In a pan that fits your air fryer, mix the eggplants with the carrots, cream and the other ingredients, toss, introduce in the air fryer and cook at 370 degrees F for 25 minutes.
2. Divide between plates and serve as a side dish.

Nutrition:

Calories: 129

Fat: 6g

Fiber: 2g

Carbs: 5g

Protein: 8g

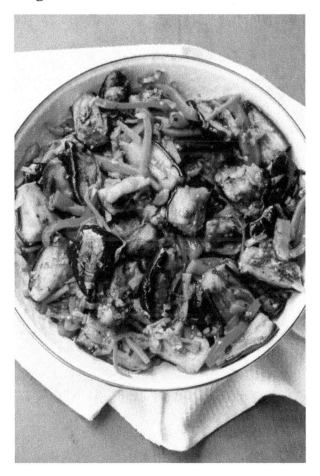

Parmesan Eggplants

Preparation time: 5 minutes

Cooking time: 20 minutes

Servings: 4

Ingredients:

- 1 pound eggplants, roughly cubed

- 1 tablespoon olive oil

- 1 teaspoon garlic powder

- 1 cup parmesan, grated

- A pinch of salt and black pepper

- Cooking spray

Directions:

1. In the air fryer's pan, mix the eggplants with the oil and the other ingredients except the parmesan and toss.

2. Sprinkle the parmesan on top, put the pan in the machine and cook at 370 degrees F for 20 minutes.

3. Divide between plates and serve as a side dish.

Nutrition:

Calories 183

Fat: 6g

Fiber: 2g

Carbs: 3g

Protein: 8g

Desserts

Chocolate Bars

Preparation Time: 10 minutes

Cooking Time: 20 minutes

Servings: 16

Ingredients:

- 15 oz cream cheese, softened

- 15 oz unsweetened dark chocolate

- 1 tsp vanilla

- 10 drops liquid stevia

Directions:

1. Grease 8-inch square dish and set aside.

2. In a saucepan dissolve chocolate over low heat.

3. Add stevia and vanilla and stir well.

4. Remove pan from heat and set aside.

5. Add cream cheese into the blender and blend until smooth.

6. Add melted chocolate mixture into the cream cheese and blend until just combined.

7. Transfer mixture into the prepared dish and spread evenly and place in the refrigerator until firm.

8. Slice and serve.

Nutrition:

Calories: 230

Fat: 24 g

Carbs: 7.5 g

Sugar: 0.1 g

Protein: 6 g

Cholesterol: 29 mg

Blueberry Muffins

Preparation Time: 15 minutes

Cooking Time: 35 minutes

Servings: 12

Ingredients:

- 2 eggs

- 1/2 cup fresh blueberries

- 1 cup heavy cream

- 2 cups almond flour

- 1/4 tsp lemon zest

- 1/2 tsp lemon extract

- 1 tsp baking powder

- 5 drops stevia

- 1/4 cup butter, melted

Directions:

1. heat the cooker to 350 F. Line muffin tin with cupcake liners and set aside.

2. Add eggs into the bowl and whisk until mix.

3. Add remaining ingredients and mix to combine.

4. Pour mixture into the prepared muffin tin and bake for 25 minutes.

5. Serve and enjoy.

Nutrition:

Calories: 190

Fat: 17 g

Carbs: 5 g

Sugar: 1 g

Protein: 5 g

Cholesterol: 55 mg

Chia Pudding

Preparation Time: 20 minutes

Cooking Time: 0 minutes

Servings: 2

Ingredients:

- 4 tbsp chia seeds

- 1 cup unsweetened coconut milk

- 1/2 cup raspberries

Directions:

1. Add raspberry and coconut milk into a blender and blend until smooth.

2. Pour mixture into the glass jar.

3. Add chia seeds in a jar and stir well.

4. Seal the jar with a lid and shake well and place in the refrigerator for 3 hours.

5. Serve chilled and enjoy.

Nutrition:

Calories: 360

Fat: 33 g

Carbs: 13 g

Sugar: 5 g

Protein: 6 g

Cholesterol: 0 mg

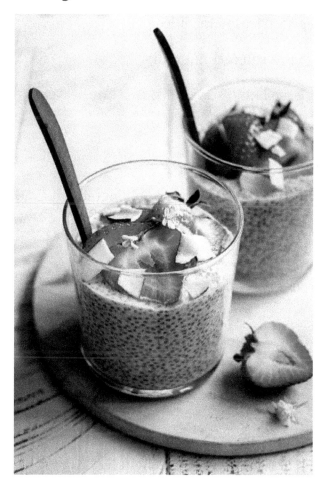

Avocado Pudding

Preparation Time: 20 minutes

Cooking Time: 0 minutes

Servings: 8

Ingredients:

- 2 ripe avocados, pitted and cut into pieces

- 1 tbsp fresh lime juice

- 14 oz can coconut milk

- 2 tsp liquid stevia

- 2 tsp vanilla

Directions:

1. Inside the blender Add all ingredients and blend until smooth.

2. Serve immediately and enjoy.

Nutrition:

Calories: 317

 Fat: 30 g

Carbs: 9 g

Sugar: 0.5 g

Protein: 3 g

Cholesterol: 0 mg

Delicious Brownie Bites

Preparation Time: 20 minutes

Cooking Time: 0 minutes

Servings: 13

Ingredients:

- 1/4 cup unsweetened chocolate chips
- 1/4 cup unsweetened cocoa powder
- 1 cup pecans, chopped
- 1/2 cup almond butter
- 1/2 tsp vanilla
- 1/4 cup monk fruit sweetener
- 1/8 tsp pink salt

Directions:

1. Add pecans, sweetener, vanilla, almond butter, cocoa powder, and salt into the food processor and process until well combined.

2. Transfer brownie mixture into the large bowl. Add chocolate chips and fold well.

3. Make small round shape balls from brownie mixture and place onto a baking tray.

4. Place in the freezer for 20 minutes.

5. Serve and enjoy.

Nutrition:

Calories: 108
Fat: 9 g
Carbs: 4 g
Sugar: 1 g
Protein: 2 g
Cholesterol: 0 mg

Lunch

Bacon Wrapped Asparagus

Preparation Time: 10 minutes

Cooking Time: 20 minutes

Servings: 2

Ingredients:

- 1/3 cup heavy whipping cream

- 2 bacon slices, precooked

- 4 small spears asparagus

- Salt, to taste

- 1 tablespoon butter

Directions:

1. Preheat the oven to 360 degrees and grease a baking sheet with butter.

2. Meanwhile, mix cream, asparagus and salt in a bowl.

3. Wrap the asparagus in bacon slices and arrange them in the baking dish.

4. Transfer the baking dish to the oven and bake for about 20 minutes.

5. Remove from the oven and serve hot.

6. Place the bacon wrapped asparagus in a dish and set aside to cool for meal prepping. Divide it in 2 containers and cover the lid. Refrigerate for about 2 days and reheat in the microwave before serving.

Nutrition:

Calories: 204

Carbs: 1.4g

Protein: 5.9g

Fat: 19.3g

Sugar: 0.5g

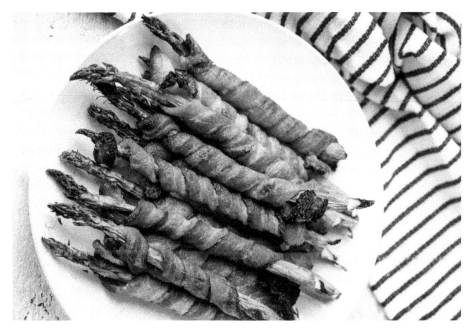

Spinach Chicken

Preparation Time: 10 minutes

Cooking Time: 10 minutes

Servings: 2

Ingredients:

- 2 garlic cloves, minced

- 2 tablespoons unsalted butter, divided

- ¼ cup parmesan cheese, shredded

- ¾ pound chicken tenders

- ¼ cup heavy cream

- 10 ounces frozen spinach, chopped

- Salt and black pepper, to taste

Directions:

1. Heat 1 tablespoon of butter in a large skillet and add chicken, salt and black pepper.

2. Cook for about 3 minutes on both sides and remove the chicken to a bowl.

3. Melt remaining butter in the skillet and add garlic, cheese, heavy cream and spinach.

4. Cook for about 2 minutes and add the chicken.

5. Cook for about 5 minutes on low heat and dish out to immediately serve.

6. Place chicken in a dish and set aside to cool for meal prepping. Divide it in 2 containers and cover them. Refrigerate for about 3 days and reheat in microwave before serving.

Nutrition:

Calories: 288

Carbs: 3.6g

Protein: 27.7g

Fat: 18.3g

Sugar: 0.3g

Lemongrass Prawns

Preparation Time: 10 minutes

Cooking Time: 15 minutes

Servings: 2

Ingredients:

- ½ red chili pepper, seeded and chopped

- 2 lemongrass stalks

- ½ pound prawns, deveined and peeled

- 6 tablespoons butter

- ¼ teaspoon smoked paprika

Directions:

1. Preheat the oven to 390 degrees and grease a baking dish.

2. Mix together red chili pepper, butter, smoked paprika and prawns in a bowl.

3. Marinate for about 2 hours and then thread the prawns on the lemongrass stalks.

4. Arrange the threaded prawns on the baking dish and transfer it in the oven.

5. Bake for about 15 minutes and dish out to serve immediately.

6. Place the prawns in a dish and set aside to cool for meal prepping. Divide it in 2 containers and close the lid. Refrigerate for about 4 days and reheat in microwave before serving.

Nutrition:

Calories: 322

Carbs: 3.8g

Protein: 34.8g

Fat: 18g

Sugar: 0.1g

Sodium: 478mg

Stuffed Mushrooms

Preparation Time: 20 minutes

Cooking Time: 25 minutes

Ingredients:

- 2 ounces bacon, crumbled

- ½ tablespoon butter

- ¼ teaspoon paprika powder

- 2 portobello mushrooms

- 1 oz cream cheese

- ¾ tablespoon fresh chives, chopped

- Salt and black pepper, to taste

Directions:

1. Preheat the oven to 400 degrees and grease a baking dish.

2. Heat butter in a skillet and add mushrooms.

3. Sauté for about 4 minutes and set aside.

4. Mix together cream cheese, chives, paprika powder, salt and black pepper in a bowl.

5. Stuff the mushrooms with this mixture and transfer on the baking dish.

6. Place in the oven and bake for about 20 minutes.

7. These mushrooms can be refrigerated for about 3 days for meal prepping and can be served with scrambled eggs.

Nutrition:

Calories: 570

Carbs: 4.6g

Protein: 19.9g

Fat: 52.8g

Sugar: 0.8g

Sodium: 1041mg

Honey Glazed Chicken Drumsticks

Preparation Time: 10 minutes

Cooking Time: 20 minutes

Servings: 2

Ingredients:

- ½ tablespoon fresh thyme, minced

- 1/8 cup Dijon mustard

- ½ tablespoon fresh rosemary, minced

- ½ tablespoon honey

- 2 chicken drumsticks

- 1 tablespoon olive oil

- Salt and black pepper, to taste

Directions:

1. Preheat the oven at 325 degrees and grease a baking dish.

2. Combine all the ingredients in a bowl except the drumsticks and mix well.

3. Add drumsticks and coat generously with the mixture.

4. Cover and refrigerate to marinate overnight.

5. Place the drumsticks in in the baking dish and transfer it in the oven.

6. Cook for about 20 minutes and dish out to immediately serve.

7. Place chicken drumsticks in a dish and set aside to cool for meal prepping. Divide it in 2 containers and cover them. Refrigerate for about 3 days and reheat in microwave before serving.

Nutrition:

Calories: 301

Carbs: 6g

Fats: 19.7g

Proteins: 4.5g

Sugar: 4.5g

Sodium: 316mg

Dinner

Zucchini Salmon Salad

Preparation Time: 5 minutes

Cooking Time: 10 minutes

Servings: 3

Ingredients:

- 2 salmon fillets

- 2 tablespoons soy sauce

- 2 zucchinis, sliced

- Salt and pepper to taste

- 2 tablespoons extra virgin olive oil

- 2 tablespoons sesame seeds

- Salt and pepper to taste

Directions:

1. Drizzle the salmon with soy sauce.

2. Heat a grill pan over medium flame. Cook salmon on the grill on each side for 2-3 minutes.

3. Season the zucchini with salt and pepper and place it on the grill as well. Cook on each side until golden.

4. Place the zucchini, salmon and the rest of the ingredients in a bowl.

5. Serve the salad fresh.

Nutrition:

Calories: 224

Fat: 19g

Protein: 18g

Carbohydrates: 0g

Pan Fried Salmon

Preparation Time: 5 minutes

Cooking Time: 20 minutes

Servings: 4

Ingredients:

- 4 salmon fillets
- Salt and pepper to taste
- 1 teaspoon dried oregano
- 1 teaspoon dried basil
- 3 tablespoons extra virgin olive oil

Directions:

1. Season the fish with salt, pepper, oregano and basil.
2. Heat the oil in a pan and place the salmon in the hot oil, with the skin facing down.
3. Fry on each side for 2 minutes until golden brown and fragrant.
4. Serve the salmon warm and fresh.

Nutrition:

Calories: 327

Fat: 25g

Protein: 36g

Carbohydrates: 0.3g

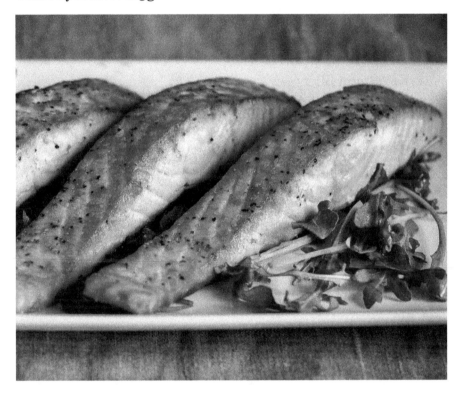

Grilled Salmon with Pineapple Salsa

Preparation Time: 5 minutes

Cooking Time: 30 minutes

Servings: 4

Ingredients:

- 4 salmon fillets
- Salt and pepper to taste
- 2 tablespoons Cajun seasoning
- 1 fresh pineapple, peeled and diced
- 1 cup cherry tomatoes, quartered
- 2 tablespoons chopped cilantro
- 2 tablespoons chopped parsley
- 1 teaspoon dried mint
- 2 tablespoons lemon juice
- 2 tablespoons extra virgin olive oil
- 1 teaspoon honey
- Salt and pepper to taste

Directions:

1. Add salt, pepper and Cajun seasoning to the fish.

2. Heat a grill pan over medium flame. Cook fish on the grill on each side for 3-4 minutes.

3. For the salsa, mix the pineapple, tomatoes, cilantro, parsley, mint, lemon juice and honey in a bowl. Season with salt and pepper.

4. Serve the grilled salmon with the pineapple salsa.

Nutrition:

Calories: 332

Fat: 12g

Protein: 34g

Carbohydrates: 0g

Chickpea Salad

Preparation Time: 5 minutes

Cooking Time: 20 minutes

Servings: 6

Ingredients:

- 1 can chickpeas, drained
- 1 fennel bulb, sliced
- 1 red onion, sliced
- 1 teaspoon dried basil
- 1 teaspoon dried oregano
- 2 tablespoons chopped parsley
- 4 garlic cloves, minced
- 2 tablespoons lemon juice
- 2 tablespoons extra virgin olive oil
- Salt and pepper to taste

Directions:

1. Combine the chickpeas, fennel, red onion, herbs, garlic, lemon juice and oil in a salad bowl.

2. Add salt and pepper and serve the salad fresh.

Nutrition:

Calories: 200

Fat: 9g

Protein: 4g

Carbohydrates: 28g

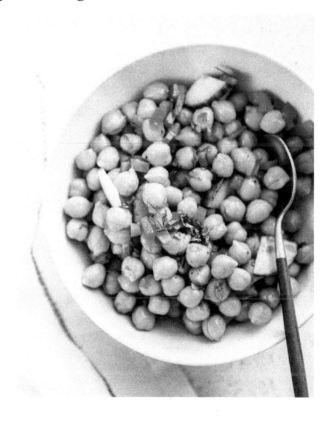

Warm Chorizo Chickpea Salad

Preparation Time: 5 minutes

Cooking Time: 20 minutes

Servings: 6

Ingredients:

- 1 tablespoon extra virgin olive oil

- 4 chorizo links, sliced

- 1 red onion, sliced

- 4 roasted red bell peppers, chopped

- 1 can chickpeas, drained

- 2 cups cherry tomatoes

- 2 tablespoons balsamic vinegar

- Salt and pepper to taste

Directions:

1. Heat the oil in a skillet and add the chorizo. Cook briefly just until fragrant then add the onion, bell peppers and chickpeas and cook for 2 additional minutes.

2. Transfer the mixture in a salad bowl then add the tomatoes, vinegar, salt and pepper.

3. Mix well and serve the salad right away.

Nutrition:

Calories: 359

Fat: 18g

Protein: 15g

Carbohydrates: 21g

Index Recipes:

CPSIA information can be obtained
at www.ICGtesting.com
Printed in the USA
BVHW051352080321
601998BV00011BA/1360